TRAUMA SOLUTIONS TAILORED FOR SENIORS

"EMPATHY, UNDERSTANDING, AND HOPE: A SENIOR-CENTERED APPROACH TO OVERCOMING ADVERSITY AND FINDING HEALING"

BLESS P. WALTON

TABLE OF CONTENTS

CHAPTER 1

NAVIGATING THE LANDSCAPE OF SENIOR TRAUMA

1.1 Understanding Trauma in Later Life

The aging process brings with it a myriad of experiences, both joyful and challenging. As we delve into the subject of senior trauma, it's crucial to first establish a comprehensive understanding of what trauma entails in the later stages of life.

Trauma for seniors can manifest in various forms, including physical, emotional, and psychological dimensions. Loss of a spouse, chronic illness, financial stress, or even the challenges associated with transitioning into assisted living can all contribute to traumatic experiences.

Unlike trauma in younger individuals, senior trauma often intersects with a lifetime of memories and experiences, making it a complex tapestry that requires careful navigation. The emotional weight of accumulated life events can magnify the impact of trauma, and understanding these unique dynamics is fundamental to tailoring effective solutions.

The physiological response to trauma also differs in seniors. Aging bodies may not rebound from stress as efficiently, potentially leading to a cascade of health issues. Chronic conditions such as arthritis or diabetes can exacerbate the effects of trauma, amplifying the need for a nuanced and comprehensive approach to recovery.

1.1.1 The Role of Past Experiences

Seniors carry with them a wealth of experiences, both positive and negative. Past traumas, unresolved issues, or even unaddressed grief from earlier life stages can resurface in later years, complicating the process of healing. Recognizing the interconnectedness of past and present experiences is crucial for developing trauma solutions that acknowledge and address the entirety of an individual's life journey.

1.1.2 Cognitive Impact of Trauma in Seniors

Understanding trauma in seniors requires an exploration of its cognitive impact. Cognitive functions may decline with age, and trauma can accelerate this process. Memory loss, difficulty concentrating, and heightened anxiety are common cognitive manifestations of senior trauma. This necessitates tailored interventions that not only address the emotional aspects but also consider cognitive well-being.

1.2 The Unique Challenges Faced by Seniors

As individuals age, they encounter a host of challenges that can contribute to the complexity of trauma experienced in later life. One prominent challenge is the loss of social connections. Seniors may face the death of friends or family members, retirement, or relocation, leading to a diminished support network. Loneliness and isolation, both significant contributors to mental health issues, can intensify the impact of trauma.

1.2.1 Health Challenges and Trauma

Physical health challenges are another facet of senior life that intersects with trauma. Chronic illnesses, pain, and mobility issues can amplify the emotional toll of traumatic events. Additionally, the fear of declining health or the loss of independence can be a source of ongoing stress for seniors, compounding the effects of trauma.

1.2.2 Financial Strain and Trauma

Financial strain is a unique challenge faced by many seniors, especially those on fixed incomes. Economic uncertainties, unexpected expenses, or inadequate retirement planning can contribute to a sense of insecurity and vulnerability. Addressing financial stress is a crucial component of holistic trauma solutions for seniors.

1.3 Breaking the Silence: Encouraging Open Conversations

One of the most formidable barriers in addressing senior trauma is the pervasive culture of silence surrounding mental health issues in older populations. Societal stigma and generational attitudes often discourage open discussions about emotional well-being, contributing to the underreporting and undertreatment of trauma among seniors.

1.3.1 Changing the Narrative: Normalizing Emotional Expression

To navigate the landscape of senior trauma effectively, it is imperative to challenge and reshape societal narratives around emotional expression in older adults. By normalizing conversations about mental health and trauma, we can create a more supportive environment that encourages seniors to seek help without fear of judgment.

1.3.2 The Importance of Storytelling and Validation

Seniors often carry untold stories, unshared grief, and unresolved emotions. Providing avenues for storytelling and validation can be a powerful therapeutic tool. By acknowledging and validating their experiences, we empower seniors to confront and process their traumas, fostering a sense of agency and control over their narratives.

Conclusion

In navigating the landscape of senior trauma, it becomes evident that a multifaceted understanding is essential. We must recognize the unique challenges faced by seniors, appreciate the interconnectedness of past and present experiences, and actively work to break the silence surrounding mental health in older populations. By doing so, we lay the foundation for effective and tailored trauma solutions that honor the resilience and wisdom inherent in the senior community. As we proceed through this exploration, subsequent chapters will delve into the empathetic approaches and customized strategies needed to guide seniors on their journey toward healing and renewal.

CHAPTER 2
THE HEART OF HEALING: EMPATHY IN TRAUMA RECOVERY

2.1 The Role of Empathy in Senior-Centered Care

Empathy serves as the cornerstone of effective trauma recovery, especially in the context of senior-centered care. As seniors navigate the complexities of trauma, the ability of caregivers, family members, and healthcare professionals to empathize becomes paramount. Empathy involves understanding and sharing the feelings of another, and in the realm of senior trauma, it is a powerful catalyst for fostering trust, connection, and healing.

2.1.1 Cultivating a Culture of Empathy

Creating a culture of empathy begins with recognizing the unique experiences of seniors and acknowledging the emotional intricacies of their journeys. It involves transcending stereotypes and preconceived notions about aging, allowing space for the individuality of each senior's narrative. This cultural shift lays the foundation for senior-centered care that is inherently empathetic.

2.1.2 The Healing Power of Empathetic Presence

Being present with empathy involves more than just understanding; it requires a genuine connection that communicates a sense of care and understanding. For seniors who may feel isolated or unheard, an empathetic presence becomes a beacon of hope, signaling that their experiences matter and are worthy of attention.

2.1.3 The Ripple Effect of Empathy

Empathy has a ripple effect, influencing not only the individual experiencing trauma but also the entire support network. Caregivers and family members who approach senior trauma with empathy create an environment that encourages healing and resilience. This ripple effect extends to the broader community, fostering a collective commitment to the well-being of seniors.

2.2 Building Trust and Connection

Trust is a fragile yet crucial element in the process of trauma recovery, particularly for seniors. Building trust involves creating an environment where seniors feel safe, respected, and understood. This trust forms the bedrock of the therapeutic relationship, enabling seniors to open up, share their experiences, and engage in the healing process.

2.2.1 Transparency and Honesty in Caregiving

Transparency and honesty are integral to building trust. Seniors need to feel that they can rely on their caregivers and healthcare providers to provide accurate information about their condition, treatment options, and the trajectory of their recovery. Clear communication fosters trust and empowers seniors to actively participate in decisions regarding their well-being.

2.2.2 Consistency in Care

Consistency in care is a key factor in building trust. Seniors benefit from routines and predictability, and caregivers who consistently provide support and empathy create a sense of reliability. This consistency helps counteract the unpredictability often associated with trauma, offering stability and security.

2.2.3 Respecting Autonomy and Choice

Respecting seniors' autonomy and choices is paramount in building trust. Trauma recovery is a deeply personal journey, and seniors should be active participants in decisions that affect their lives. Empowering them to make choices, even in the small details of their care, reinforces their sense of agency and builds trust in the caregiving relationship.

2.3 Empathetic Listening: A Gateway to Understanding

Listening with empathy is an art that transcends hearing words; it involves understanding the emotions, fears, and hopes behind those words. For seniors navigating trauma, empathetic listening becomes a gateway to understanding their unique experiences and perspectives.

2.3.1 Creating Safe Spaces for Expression

Seniors need safe spaces to express their thoughts and emotions without fear of judgment. Empathetic listening involves creating an environment where seniors feel heard, validated, and understood. This safe space is essential for seniors to process their trauma and begin the journey toward healing.

2.3.2 Non-Verbal Cues and Understanding Emotion

Understanding goes beyond words; it involves attuning to non-verbal cues and recognizing the emotional undertones of communication. Many seniors may struggle to articulate their feelings verbally, making non-verbal communication an essential aspect of empathetic listening. Caregivers and healthcare professionals must be attuned to facial expressions, body language, and other subtle cues.

2.3.3 Reflective Listening and Validation

Reflective listening is a technique that involves summarizing and reflecting back what the speaker has expressed. This not only demonstrates active engagement but also provides an opportunity for clarification and validation. Seniors benefit from knowing that their experiences are acknowledged and that their feelings are valid.

Conclusion

In the heart of healing lies empathy—a force that transcends understanding and extends into the realms of connection, trust, and compassionate listening. As we navigate the landscape of senior trauma, it is crucial to recognize the pivotal role of empathy in providing senior-centered care.

Building trust, fostering connection, and engaging in empathetic listening create a foundation for trauma recovery that honors the individuality and resilience of seniors. In the subsequent chapters, we will explore tailored strategies and holistic approaches that leverage the power of empathy to guide

seniors on their path to healing and renewal.

CHAPTER 3

TAILORING SOLUTIONS: CUSTOMIZED APPROACHES FOR SENIORS

3.1 Holistic Wellness for Aging Bodies and Minds

Addressing trauma in seniors requires a holistic approach that considers the interconnectedness of physical, emotional, and mental well-being. Holistic wellness for aging bodies and minds involves recognizing that the impact of trauma extends beyond the emotional realm, influencing overall health and quality of life.

3.1.1 Physical Activity and Seniors: A Vital Connection

Physical activity plays a crucial role in holistic wellness for seniors. Regular exercise not only contributes to physical health but also has profound effects on mental and emotional well-being. Tailoring exercise programs to seniors' abilities and preferences fosters a sense of accomplishment and helps alleviate symptoms of trauma such as anxiety and depression.

3.1.2 Nutrition as a Foundation for Healing

Nutrition is a key component of holistic wellness. Seniors recovering from trauma may experience changes in appetite, dietary habits, or nutritional deficiencies. Crafting personalized nutrition plans that address these specific needs not only supports physical recovery but also contributes to mental clarity and emotional stability.

3.1.3 Mind-Body Practices for Emotional Resilience

Holistic wellness involves the integration of mind-body practices that promote emotional resilience. Practices such as meditation, yoga, and tai chi have been shown to reduce stress, improve mood, and enhance overall well-being. Tailoring these practices to the unique needs and preferences of seniors provides a holistic approach to trauma recovery.

3.2 Crafting Individualized Trauma Recovery Plans

No two individuals experience trauma in the same way, and seniors, with their diverse life experiences, require personalized and flexible approaches to trauma recovery. Crafting individualized trauma recovery plans involves a collaborative process that takes into account the unique strengths, challenges, and preferences of each senior.

3.2.1 Assessment and Collaboration

The first step in crafting an individualized trauma recovery plan is a comprehensive assessment. This involves understanding the senior's history, identifying specific trauma triggers, and assessing current mental and physical health. Collaboration with the senior, caregivers, and healthcare professionals ensures that the plan is informed by multiple perspectives and tailored to the individual's needs.

3.2.2 Setting Realistic Goals and Milestones

Setting realistic and achievable goals is a key component of individualized trauma recovery plans. Seniors may have specific aspirations related to their recovery, whether it's improving social connections, managing symptoms of anxiety, or regaining a sense of purpose. Tailoring goals to align with the senior's priorities ensures that the recovery plan is meaningful and motivating.

3.2.3 Flexibility and Adaptability

Trauma recovery is a dynamic process, and an individualized plan must be flexible and adaptable. Seniors may encounter unexpected challenges or changes in their circumstances, and the recovery plan should evolve to address these shifts. Regular reassessment and adjustments ensure that the plan remains relevant and supportive throughout the recovery journey.

3.3 Integrating Complementary Therapies for Lasting Healing

Complementary therapies, when integrated into trauma recovery plans, offer additional tools for seniors to address the emotional and physical aspects of their experiences. These therapies, ranging from creative arts to mindfulness practices, provide avenues for expression, self-discovery, and relaxation.

3.3.1 Art and Music Therapy: Creative Expression for Healing

Creative arts therapies, such as art and music therapy, offer seniors alternative ways to express and process their emotions. Engaging in artistic activities provides a non-verbal outlet for trauma-related feelings, fostering a sense of empowerment and creativity. These therapies can be tailored to accommodate varying levels of physical ability and cognitive function.

3.3.2   Mindfulness   and   Meditation: Cultivating Presence

Mindfulness and meditation practices are powerful tools for seniors navigating trauma. Tailored mindfulness programs can help seniors cultivate presence, manage stress, and develop coping strategies. These practices can be adapted to suit individual preferences, whether through guided meditation sessions, mindful breathing exercises, or nature-based contemplation.

3.3.3 Animal-Assisted Therapy: Fostering Connection

Creature-helped treatment includes cooperation with prepared creatures to advance close to home prosperity. For seniors, especially those experiencing isolation or loneliness, integrating animal-assisted therapy into recovery plans can foster a sense of connection and companionship. Tailoring these interactions to accommodate seniors' physical abilities ensures a positive and enriching experience.

Conclusion

Tailoring solutions for senior trauma involves a holistic and individualized approach that recognizes the interconnectedness of physical, emotional, and mental well-being. By promoting holistic wellness through physical activity, nutrition, and mind-body practices, seniors can embark on a comprehensive journey toward healing. Crafting individualized trauma recovery plans ensures that the unique needs and preferences of each senior are considered, fostering a sense of agency and purpose.

Integrating complementary therapies provides additional avenues for expression and healing, offering seniors a diverse toolkit for lasting well-being. In the following chapters, we will delve deeper into the empathetic and personalized strategies that form the heart of trauma solutions tailored for seniors.

CHAPTER 4

CULTIVATING HOPE: STRATEGIES FOR SENIORS' RESILIENCE

4.1 The Power of Positive Aging

Positive aging is a philosophy that emphasizes the potential for growth, fulfillment, and contribution in the later stages of life. Cultivating hope through the lens of positive aging recognizes that seniors possess unique strengths, wisdom, and resilience that can be harnessed for trauma recovery.

4.1.1 Embracing Life Transitions

Positive aging involves embracing life transitions as opportunities for growth rather than as obstacles. Whether it's retirement, relocation, or the loss of a loved one, seniors can navigate these changes with a positive mindset that focuses on the possibilities inherent in each new chapter of life. Recognizing and celebrating the value of these transitions contributes to a sense of purpose and hope.

4.1.2 Fostering a Positive Self-Image

Promoting a positive self-image is essential for seniors recovering from trauma. Negative self-perceptions can hinder resilience and exacerbate the impact of traumatic experiences. Encouraging seniors to recognize and celebrate their accomplishments, skills, and unique qualities fosters a positive self-image that serves as a foundation for hope and resilience.

4.1.3 Engaging in Meaningful Activities

Positive aging is enriched by engaging in activities that bring joy, meaning, and a sense of accomplishment. Tailoring activities to align with seniors' interests and abilities fosters a positive and hopeful outlook. Whether it's pursuing hobbies, volunteering, or connecting with others, meaningful activities contribute to a fulfilling and purpose-driven life.

4.2 Finding Hope Amidst Adversity

In the face of trauma, finding hope becomes a transformative journey that requires acknowledging challenges while actively seeking positive elements. Seniors navigating adversity can draw upon various strategies to discover and nurture hope in their lives.

4.2.1 Cultivating Gratitude

Practicing gratitude is a powerful tool for finding hope amidst adversity. Seniors can develop a gratitude practice by reflecting on positive aspects of their lives, acknowledging small victories, and expressing appreciation for the support they receive. Cultivating gratitude shifts focus from challenges to blessings, fostering a hopeful perspective.

4.2.2 Connecting with Supportive Communities

Social connections are integral to finding hope. Seniors benefit from connecting with supportive communities, whether through friendships, support groups, or social organizations. These connections provide a network of understanding and encouragement, creating a sense of belonging and hope in times of adversity.

4.2.3 Setting Realistic Expectations

Setting realistic expectations is crucial for seniors navigating trauma. By acknowledging and accepting limitations while recognizing possibilities, seniors can maintain a hopeful outlook. Setting achievable goals, celebrating progress, and adapting to changing circumstances contribute to a sense of agency and hopefulness.

4.3 Building a Resilient Mindset for Senior Well-being

Resilience is the capacity to bounce back from adversity, and building a resilient mindset is a key component of senior well-being. Cultivating resilience involves developing coping strategies, fostering adaptability, and nurturing a positive outlook on life.

4.3.1 Developing Coping Strategies

Seniors can build resilience by developing effective coping strategies to manage stress and adversity. These strategies may include mindfulness practices, problem-solving skills, and seeking support when needed. Tailoring coping mechanisms to align with individual preferences and strengths enhances their effectiveness in promoting resilience.

4.3.2 Fostering Adaptability

Adaptability is a hallmark of resilience. Seniors can cultivate adaptability by embracing change, developing flexible thinking, and adjusting to new circumstances. Navigating trauma often requires adapting to evolving emotions, physical abilities, and life circumstances. Fostering adaptability contributes to a resilient mindset that empowers seniors to face challenges with confidence.

4.3.3 Nurturing a Positive Outlook on Aging

A positive outlook on aging is a potent factor in resilience. Seniors who view aging as a time of continued growth, learning, and possibilities are more likely to navigate trauma with resilience. Nurturing a positive perspective involves challenging ageist stereotypes, embracing the inherent value of aging, and recognizing the strength that comes with experience.

Conclusion

Cultivating hope and resilience is an essential aspect of senior trauma recovery. By embracing the power of positive aging, finding hope amidst adversity, and building a resilient mindset, seniors can navigate the challenges of trauma with strength and purpose.

These strategies not only contribute to emotional well-being but also empower seniors to actively engage in their recovery journey. In the subsequent chapters, we will explore further empathetic approaches and tailored solutions that continue to guide seniors on the path to healing and renewal.

CHAPTER 5

A JOURNEY TO RENEWAL: THRIVING AFTER TRAUMA

5.1 Celebrating Small Victories in Senior Trauma Recovery

In the journey to renewal after trauma, celebrating small victories becomes a vital component of fostering resilience and well-being among seniors. Small victories, often overlooked, hold the power to instill a sense of accomplishment, boost self-esteem, and provide momentum for continued progress.

5.1.1 Recognizing the Significance of Small Wins

Seniors recovering from trauma may face various challenges, and acknowledging the significance of small victories is crucial.

Whether it's completing a daily task, engaging in a new activity, or expressing emotions, each achievement contributes to the overall trajectory of recovery. Recognizing and celebrating these small wins creates a positive feedback loop, reinforcing the belief in one's ability to overcome adversity.

5.1.2 Setting Realistic Milestones

Setting realistic milestones aligns with the concept of celebrating small victories. Seniors, in collaboration with caregivers and healthcare professionals, can establish achievable goals that reflect their unique needs and aspirations. These milestones serve as stepping stones on the path to renewal, providing motivation and a sense of progress.

5.1.3 Fostering a Growth Mindset

Cultivating a growth mindset involves viewing challenges as opportunities for learning and growth. Seniors can embrace the idea that abilities and skills can be developed over time, fostering resilience in the face of trauma. Celebrating small victories becomes a natural outcome of a growth mindset, as each step forward is seen as a testament to one's capacity for positive change.

5.2 Connecting with Community: The Role of Social Support

Social support is a powerful force in senior trauma recovery, providing a network of understanding, encouragement, and companionship. Connecting with community, whether through existing relationships or by forging new connections, enhances the overall well-being of seniors on their journey to renewal.

5.2.1 The Impact of Social Isolation on Trauma Recovery

Social isolation can significantly impact seniors recovering from trauma. Feelings of loneliness and a lack of social connections may exacerbate the emotional toll of trauma. Recognizing the importance of social support and actively seeking connection is fundamental to fostering a supportive community.

5.2.2 Building and Strengthening Relationships

Seniors benefit from building and strengthening relationships with family, friends, and peers. Caregivers and healthcare professionals play a pivotal role in facilitating these connections by creating opportunities for social interaction. Group activities, support networks, and community events contribute to a sense of belonging and shared experiences.

5.2.3 Encouraging Open Communication

Open communication is key to meaningful connections. Seniors should be encouraged to express their thoughts, feelings, and needs, fostering a sense of trust and understanding within their social circles. Caregivers and community members who actively listen and validate seniors' experiences contribute to a supportive environment that promotes renewal after trauma.

5.3 Embracing the Golden Years with Renewed Purpose

As seniors navigate trauma recovery, embracing the golden years with renewed purpose becomes a transformative goal. Finding meaning, pursuing passions, and contributing to the community are essential elements that can redefine the senior experience and foster a sense of fulfillment.

5.3.1 Rediscovering Passions and Hobbies

Seniors often find renewal by rediscovering passions and hobbies that bring joy and fulfillment. Whether it's engaging in creative arts, gardening, or lifelong learning, reconnecting with activities that resonate with personal interests contributes to a sense of purpose and meaning.

5.3.2 Volunteerism and Community Engagement

Engaging in volunteerism and community activities allows seniors to contribute their time and skills, fostering a sense of purpose and connection. By actively participating in initiatives that align with their values, seniors can experience the fulfillment that comes from making a positive impact on the lives of others.

5.3.3 Creating a Personal Legacy

As seniors embrace the golden years, the concept of creating a personal legacy takes on significance. This involves reflecting on life experiences, sharing wisdom with younger generations, and leaving a positive imprint on the community. The act of creating a legacy provides a sense of continuity and purpose, transcending the challenges of trauma.

Conclusion

Chapter 5 explores the transformative journey to renewal after trauma for seniors. By celebrating small victories, connecting with community, and embracing the golden years with renewed purpose, seniors can navigate the complexities of trauma recovery with resilience and optimism.

The integration of these strategies not only contributes to emotional well-being but also empowers seniors to redefine their experiences and find meaning in the later stages of life. As we conclude this exploration, it becomes evident that renewal is not only a destination but a continuous process—one that unfolds through the celebration of victories, the strength of social connections, and the discovery of purpose in the golden years.

CONCLUSION

FOSTERING A CULTURE OF EMPATHY AND RESILIENCE

Reflecting on the Senior-Centered Approach

The journey through the chapters of "Trauma Solutions Tailored for Seniors: Empathy, Understanding, and Hope" has been a comprehensive exploration of the unique challenges faced by seniors in the realm of trauma and the nuanced strategies essential for their recovery. At the core of this exploration is the senior-centered approach, a philosophy that recognizes the individuality, experiences, and resilience of the aging population.

Reflecting on the senior-centered approach, it becomes evident that empathy is the guiding force. Empathy, the ability to understand and share the feelings of another, forms the bedrock of effective trauma solutions.

From understanding trauma in later life to building trust, fostering connection, and engaging in empathetic listening, the senior-centered approach places the emotional well-being of seniors at its forefront. It challenges societal norms and encourages open conversations about mental health, breaking the silence that often surrounds the emotional experiences of older individuals.

The senior-centered approach extends to the tailoring of solutions, recognizing that one size does not fit all. Seniors are a diverse group with varied life experiences, strengths, and challenges. Holistic wellness, individualized trauma recovery plans, and the integration of complementary therapies ensure that solutions are crafted to address the interconnected dimensions of physical, emotional, and mental well-being. This tailored approach respects the autonomy and choices of seniors, empowering them to actively participate in their healing journey.

Inspiring Lasting Trauma Solutions for the Aging Generation

As we conclude this exploration, the focus shifts to inspiring lasting trauma solutions for the aging generation. The trajectory of senior trauma recovery extends beyond immediate interventions; it involves fostering a culture of empathy and resilience that permeates every facet of senior care and support.

1. Cultivating a Culture of Empathy

Inspiring lasting trauma solutions begins with cultivating a culture of empathy—a culture that values and prioritizes the emotional well-being of seniors. This involves challenging ageist stereotypes and recognizing the strength and resilience inherent in aging individuals. By promoting empathy, we create an environment where seniors feel heard, understood, and supported in their unique journeys.

2. Empowering Caregivers and Healthcare Professionals

The lasting impact of trauma solutions relies on the empowerment of caregivers and healthcare professionals. Training programs that emphasize the importance of empathy, active listening, and tailored care for seniors equip professionals with the skills needed to provide effective support. The dissemination of trauma-informed practices ensures that senior care becomes a holistic and empathetic endeavor.

3. Integrating Trauma Solutions into Healthcare Systems

Lasting trauma solutions require the integration of trauma-informed care into healthcare systems. This involves creating protocols and practices that consider the emotional well-being of seniors in various healthcare settings. From routine check-ups to specialized care, a trauma-informed approach ensures that the unique needs of seniors are consistently addressed.

4. Promoting Research and Innovation

Inspiring lasting trauma solutions involves an ongoing commitment to research and innovation. Understanding the evolving needs of the aging population and exploring new therapeutic modalities contribute to the advancement of trauma solutions. By staying abreast of emerging knowledge and continuously refining approaches, we ensure that seniors receive the most effective and cutting-edge care.

5. Advocating for Mental Health in Aging

Advocacy plays a pivotal role in inspiring lasting trauma solutions. By advocating for mental health awareness, reducing stigma, and influencing policy changes, we create a societal landscape that prioritizes the emotional well-being of seniors. This advocacy extends to the allocation of resources for mental health services tailored to the aging population.

A Call to Action

As we conclude our journey through the realms of senior-centered trauma solutions, it is a call to action for caregivers, healthcare professionals, policymakers, and society as a whole. Fostering a culture of empathy and resilience requires collective effort and a commitment to valuing the experiences and emotional needs of seniors.

It is a call to empower the aging generation by providing them with the tools, support, and understanding needed for their trauma recovery. It is a call to challenge societal norms, break down barriers to mental health discussions, and create an environment where seniors can age with dignity, purpose, and resilience.

In inspiring lasting trauma solutions for the aging generation, we not only enhance the quality of life for individuals but also contribute to a more compassionate and empathetic society. The journey to renewal after trauma is ongoing, and by fostering a culture that embraces empathy and resilience, we pave the way for seniors to thrive in the later stages of life.